I0083602

Dash Diet

The Most Recent Dash Cookbook With Simple And Delectable Low Sodium Recipes For Weight Loss And Heart Health

(Day Heart-Healthy Dietary Plan To Kick-Start Your Diet)

Surinder Woolley

TABLE OF CONTENT

Introduction

This program's acronym is DASH for Dietary Approaches to Stop Hypertension. The DASH diet (hypertension) is a low-fat, high-fiber diet that can be used to treat or prevent hypertension.

The DASH diet includes potassium-, calcium-, and magnesium-rich foods. By consuming these nutrients, blood pressure can be managed. On the regimen, foods high in salt, saturated fat, and added sugars are restricted.

According to multiple studies, the DASH diet can reduce blood pressure within two weeks. Diet can also reduce low-density lipoprotein cholesterol (LDL or "bad") levels. Two major risk factors for heart disease and stroke are hypertension and elevated LDL cholesterol levels.

Dietary Counsel

Both dinners ought to include vegetables.

Fruit can be consumed with meals or as a nutritious refreshment. Conserving and dehydrating fruits is convenient, but make sure they do not contain sugar.

Use half as much butter, margarine, or salad dressing and substitute with low-fat or fat-free condiments.

• Consume low-fat or nonfat dairy products in place of full-fat or cream products.

Every day, you should consume no more than six ounces of flesh. Make a portion of your diet plant-based.

You should consume more vegetables and beans.

Nuts, raisins, low-fat and fat-free yogurt, and frozen yogurt are all nutritious alternatives to potato crisps and sweets. Raw vegetables and unsalted popcorn are also excellent options.

By perusing food labels, you can reduce your sodium intake.

The DASH Diet must be followed strictly.

The DASH diet suggests the following:

7 to 8 servings of grains daily

8 -10 daily servings of vegetables

8 -10 portions of fruit daily

Aim for two to three daily servings of low-fat or fat-free dairy products.

Meat, poultry, and fish should not exceed two servings per day.

At least four to five portions of nuts, seeds, and dry legumes per week.

2-6 servings of lipids and oils per day are recommended.

Try to consume no more than five treats per week.

There is controversy regarding the size of a serving.

When attempting to adhere to a healthy eating plan, knowing how much of a particular product constitutes one serving is useful information. The following is a one-person serving size:

- 1 cup of cooked rice or pasta • bread, a single slice • 2 cup of unprocessed vegetables or fruits.

- a half-cup of cooked vegetables or fruit • one cup of milk

- One-tenth of a teaspoon of olive oil (or any other oil); • Three ounces of cooked meat; • Three ounces of tofu.

Prospective Advantages

Two potential benefits of the DASH diet, which lowers blood pressure, are weight loss and reduced cancer risk.

Because of this, you should not place too much faith in DASH's capacity to promote weight loss on its own. Weight loss may be a mere benefit.

Diet has numerous effects on the human organism.

Who are the prospective recipients?

Dietary Approach to Stop Hypertension (DASH) can lower: • systolic blood pressure

• blood sugar levels

Triglycerides of the blood

LDL stands for lipoprotein low-density lipoprotein.

An elevated insulin resistance

In addition to these symptoms, metabolic syndrome also includes obesity, type 2 diabetes, and an increased risk of cardiac disease.

After following the DASH diet for eight weeks, researchers discovered that the health of both individuals with and without metabolic syndrome improved significantly.

According to the results, the average number of participants was:

In persons with metabolic disorders, systolic blood pressure decreased by 8 ,9 mm Hg, and diastolic blood pressure decreased by 2 ,9 mm Hg.

The systolic and diastolic blood pressures of those without metabolic syndrome decreased by 10 .2% and 2.9%, respectively.

If you have metabolic syndrome, DASH may help you reduce your blood pressure. In addition, research suggests that it may reduce the risk of colorectal cancer and generally increase longevity.

The National Kidney Foundation recommends DASH for those with kidney disease.

What are some foods that lower blood sugar levels?

Knowing a person's systolic blood pressure

The systolic pressure is measured when the heart is actively flowing blood, while the diastolic pressure is measured between heartbeats. A reading of 2

20/80 mm Hg indicates systolic and diastolic blood pressures of 2 20/80 mm Hg.

Current American College of Cardiology guidelines regarding blood pressure state:

Below 2 20/80 millimeters of mercury is normal blood pressure.

Systolic pressure is between 2 20 and 2 29 mm Hg, and diastolic pressure is below 80 mm Hg.

Stage 2 blood pressure readings are 2 6 0-2 6 9 mmHg and 80-89 mmHg, respectively.

Stage 2 hypertension: 2 8 0 systolic and/or 90 diastolic or higher.

Diastolic is greater than 2 20, and systolic is greater than 2 80.

Yes, I intend to lose weight.

Weight loss is possible but not required on the DASH diet. If one desires to lose weight, the National Heart, Lung, and Blood Institute (NHLBI) suggests a gradual reduction in caloric intake.

Other DASH weight loss recommendations include: eating several small meals per day; consuming more fruits, vegetables, and whole grains in lieu of red meat.

Instead of candy and crackers, snack on fruits and vegetables.

The National Institute of Diabetes, Digestive, and Kidney Diseases body mass index calculator.

- adhering to the DASH diet of the NHLBI, which includes a calorie chart

Dietary types A and B of DASH

The DASH diet easy come in both low-calorie and high-calorie varieties.

The DASH diet recommends a sodium intake of up to 2,6 00 milligrams (mg) per day.

On this regimen, 2 ,10 00 mg of sodium is permitted daily.

Because many individuals in the United States consume more than 6 ,600 mg of sodium per day, each of the DASH diets emphasizes reducing sodium intake.

One clinical trial revealed that combining the DASH diet with a limited sodium intake had a greater effect on blood pressure than either one alone.

People should consume more potassium-rich foods while reducing their sodium intake. Potassium's ability to dilate blood vessels can lead to a reduction in blood pressure. For optimal health and wellbeing, it is essential to consume an adequate amount of potassium daily.

Potassium-rich foods include dried fruit such as dates, raisins, apricots, etc., legumes such as lentils and kidney beans, squash, potatoes, orange juice, bananas, and dried fruit.

Dried apricots are an exceptional source of the mineral potassium. A cup of prepared lentils provides approximately 22 % of the daily fiber requirement.

A diet founded on the Mediterranean way of life may also benefit the heart and overall health.

What is permissible to consume

The DASH diet emphasizes seasonal fruits and vegetables, low-fat dairy products, and whole grains.

• complete cereals

Additionally, poultry and fish are included in this category.

Moderate red meat, cholesterol, and sugar consumption

It is low in total fat, saturated fat, and cholesterol.

On average, a person observing a DASH diet of 2,000 calories per day might consume the following foods:

This recipe contains 6–8 servings of grains. Examples include pasta and rice, as well as cereals and breads. Whole wheat bread, pasta, rice, and cereal all constitute a single serving. One ounce of powdered cereal is also acceptable.

Four to five servings of vegetables, including vegetables rich in fiber and vitamins. Broccoli, sweet potatoes, and other vegetables that thrive in the soil come to mind. One serving consists of half a cup of raw or cooked vegetables, or one cup of fresh, green, leafy vegetables.

Four to five servings of fruit are recommended daily. These contain fiber, magnesium, potassium, and numerous vitamins and minerals. A half-cup serving can contain fresh, canned, or frozen fruit, or one medium-sized piece of raw fruit.

Low-fat or fat-free dairy product Approximately two to three servings: These nutrients are abundant in both vitamin D and calcium. 2 cup of yogurt, skim milk, or milk with less than 2 % fat can all be counted as one serving.

Six 2 -ounce portions of fish, poultry, or lean meat. Red meat is high in protein, B vitamins, zinc, iron, and other essential nutrients; therefore, those following the DASH diet should limit their consumption. This meal can contain cooked, skinless poultry, lean meat or seafood, one egg, and one ounce of tuna packed in water with no added sodium.

8 –10 ounces of nuts, seeds, and legumes per day. These foods contain

essential nutrients such as protein and potassium. Examples of legumes include sunflower seeds, beans, peas, lentils, almonds, peanuts, and pistachios.

2 to 6 portions of healthful fats and oils. In addition to aiding in the absorption of vitamins and other nutrients, fat also contributes to the maintenance of the immune system. Two tablespoons of margarine, low-fat mayonnaise, or a light salad condiment may be included in one serving.

Up to five servings of desserts per week. Although the DASH diet emphasizes limiting sweets, it does not explicitly prohibit them. One serving consists of one cup of lemonade, one-half cup of sorbet, one tablespoon of sugar, marmalade, or jelly, and one-half cup of ice cream.

To adhere to the DASH diet, men and women should consume no more than two alcoholic beverages per day, while women should consume no more than one.

Depending on their age, gender, and level of activity, each individual will have distinct caloric requirements.

A 10 2 -year-old woman who is not very active requires no more than 2 ,600 calories per day, while a 210 -year-old man who is exceedingly active requires 6 ,000 calories per day.

Chapter 1: Plant Based Foods

The emphasis on plant-based nutrition is not an error. The DASH diet expressly excludes creature items, as they are somejust thing we typically enjoy without comprehension. The dairy and livestock industry is one of the largest in the country; it is financed and generates substantial revenue by claiming that the product is essential for health. In light of this, we frequently use "our body needs it" as an excuse to consume meat and dairy. Actually, most processed meats and dairy are unhealthy and loaded with sodium. Similarly, we are completely unaware that a serving is a quarter of the size we are acclimated to seeing.

Plant-based food sources make it easier to consume more (somejust thing we're typically guilty of) while still enjoying a delicious meal. Those who consume a diet rich in plant-based foods have a 20% reduced risk of developing coronary disease and a 27% lower risk of dying from cardiovascular infection, according to research. They are also less likely to experience the adverse effects of hypertension. It is debatable whether this risk is specifically related to the reduced consumption of these products or whether it is the result of the decreased sodium and chemical ingestion that results from eliminating them.

Probably your next query will be, but what about protein and calcium? Did you know that the majority of plant foods contain both? The majority of plant foods contain more protein than meat when consumed in appropriate portions. The same can be said regarding calcium and leafy green vegetables. Many nut milks contain more calcium than cow's milk, but have less lactose and no cholesterol. The majority of plant-based eaters report feeling more satisfied and satiated after a meal. While it may seem absurd to eliminate all meat and dairy, the DASH diet does not require you to do so. You are permitted to consume a limited amount of meat and dairy, so you are required to adhere to the diet. It is also feasible in the long term to adopt the DASH vegan diet. This is perhaps the greatest advantage of this diet over others; practically nojust thing is forbidden as long as it is consumed in moderation.

DASH & Exercise

In addition to dietary restrictions, both the original DASH and the weight loss adaptation encourage exercise. Even in modest amounts, staying active has numerous benefits for the body. Strolling is regarded as possibly the best form of exercise due to its minimal impact and efficiency. The only costs associated with walking are quality footwear and time. You can walk virtually everywhere. This is especially crucial if you are not accustomed to exercising, as it is not as taxing on the body as running or HIIT. Inquire with your primary care physician prior to beginning an exercise regimen, as your pulse may reveal concealed health problems that could be exacerbated by physical activity.

It has been demonstrated that moderate exercise improves both circulatory tension and mental health, which is another reason you should incorporate it just into your DASH plan. Exercise is a standard adjustment to most lifestyles and should fit in effectively. Studies have demonstrated that obese adults who followed the DASH diet had improved health, greater dissemination, and greater weight loss than those who followed the diet alone.

Now that you are aware of what you are consuming, you can examine how the DASH diet fits just into nutritional categories. All DASH plans follow comparative food groupings, so this applies whether you are following the first or weight loss iteration.

Food Classes

Grains:

Grains are the most common source of processed goods in the average diet. Choose whole-grain, steel-cut, and high-fiber options whenever possible. Cereals, rice, pasta, and bread are all grain sources, but you can also add amaranth and quinoa to your diet for variety. Whole grains metabolize more slowly in the body and contain more vitamins and minerals because they are not refined. Any white foods, such as white rice, white bread, and white pasta, typically have these nutrients removed and either replaced with chemical substitutes or eliminated entirely. The fiber in these foods helps you feel satiated for longer and can also aid in digestive regulation.

Vegetables:

Crucial to the DASH diet are dark leafy greens, colorful vegetables, and cruciferous vegetables such as broccoli. It is recommended that you consume as many of these as possible because they are low in cholesterol, high in fiber, and rich in essential nutrients for a healthy diet. The majority of vegetables are rich in fiber and nutrients, but there are a few that should be avoided due to their high carbohydrate content. Potatoes are an excellent example of this. The reason starch should be avoided is because it is converted just into sugar by the body, so even if you don't add sugar to your diet, you may consume an excessive amount of sugar by consuming bland foods.

The manner in which you easy cook your vegetables has a substantial impact on whether or not they are DASH-friendly. Given that the diet emphasizes low-fat foods, singing is a poor choice. Due to the manner in which they are prepared, tempura vegetables, fries, singed tomatoes, and hash browns should be avoided on a diet. Some vegetable condiments should also be scrutinized because of the sodium content. If you intend to prepare a sauce for your vegetables, consider preparing it yourself to reduce the fat and sodium content.

Fruits: Fruits are also high in fiber and nutrient density, but they are also high in natural carbohydrates. Due to this, natural products should be avoided during stage one and used with caution during stage two. A few organic products contain more sugar than others, and those that contain more fiber can offset some of the sugar. Apples, pears, and melons are all examples of this because they have high fructose levels but high fiber content. Avocados should be avoided on the DASH diet because they are typically rich in fat. You'll also want to avoid dried fruits unless you make them yourself, as store-bought dried fruits are frequently sugar-coated prior to drying.

Choose canned organic foods that contain water or their own contents as a liquid to reduce the amount of added sugar. Additionally, you can save the juice and use it sparingly to flavor water or in cookery.

Dairy:

Although dairy is rich in calcium and protein, it should be consumed with moderation when following the DASH diet. Depending on the product, dairy is high in lactose and can also be high in lipids and sodium. Choose low-fat or non-fat dairy, being mindful of the sugar content, as these will still be satisfying but have fewer calories. Additionally, dairy is a good source of vitamin D, B vitamins, and vitamin A. Yogurts and processed cheeses should be examined for ingredients first, as they frequently contain added substances that push them too far just into the sodium and sugar categories to merit the benefits.

Legumes, Nuts, and Seeds

Not all vegetables are regarded as vegetables, some are viewed as vegetables. Beans are commonly considered a vegetable but are in fact vegetables, and the same holds true for soy products. A significant portion of them are also high in fiber and protein, making them an optimal option for the DASH diet. If they are combined with whole cereals, the result is astoundingly improved. Vegetables are an excellent substitute for meat and dairy when attempting to lose weight. Nuts and seeds are also high in protein and therefore beneficial. Obtain a version of nuts that is unsalted and less processed in order to reduce sodium intake. Because nuts and seeds are such calorie-dense foods, you will also need to consider the portion size.

Meat, Fish, Poultry, and Eggs:

As we have heard, we frequently consume a greater quantity of these liquid food sources than solid ones. To be able to recollect these items for your diet without becoming overly indulgent, it is essential to learn the serving sizes of these foods. Most animal products are extremely high in cholesterol and saturated fat, so it is best to choose slender options whenever possible. In general, fish will be reduced in fat but higher in cholesterol. Here are some serving size suggestions:

6 oz. of seafood

6 oz chicken bosom 6 eggs

6 oz lean flesh

When selecting meats, try to avoid store-bought processed meats, which are typically loaded with added substances and sodium; even the reduced sodium varieties can be extremely high. Consider purchasing a home meat slicer or sparingly slicing additional meat for use on sandwiches. Choose grass-fed products because they are superior and less likely to contain added substances.

Fats:

We've come to realize that there are healthy fats and unhealthy fats, but the 2 980s rhetoric that all fat is evil still haunts us. We frequently find "fat-free" foods appealing, despite the fact that the low-fat version contains substantially more sugar to compensate for the loss of flavor. Similarly, you will find fat concealed in foods such as salad dressings and marinades, which you may not count. On the DASH diet, some fats are unquestionably healthier than others. You should avoid fats that have been extensively processed, such as vegetable oil and the majority of frying oils. Choose grass-fed butter and olive oil instead. Avoid margarine, shortening, and trans-fat-containing foods. Synthetic trans fats have been linked to circulatory disorders. Many commercial bakery products are laden with fats to enhance their flavor; therefore, it is crucial to examine the list of ingredients. In many diets, potato chips and certain peanut butters are also deceptive sources of fat.

Chapter 3: The Dash Diet: Healthy Eating For Blood Pressure Control

In general, there is already an abundance of food, and you can help yourself by avoiding the common foods that people with high blood pressure should routinely avoid. Diet is the foundation of wellness. In fact, consuming healthful foods reduces a variety of health issues. This includes hypertension (high blood pressure). The proper diet can reduce blood pressure. Your physician may recommend the DASH diet to help reduce your hypertension and cholesterol levels.

The DASH diet addresses the leading causes of elevated blood pressure on multiple fronts. Reduced sodium intake is the most apparent antihypertensive feature of the DASH diet.

When the body contains excessive sodium, the blood accumulates more water, which raises the blood vessel pressure. Then, this pressure causes your arteries and vessels to enlarge and constrict, thereby reducing the available space for blood flow. Consequently, this reduces the quantity of blood absorbed by various body parts with each heartbeat. By decreasing sodium ingestion, the blood can be returned to its normal water content, thereby relieving the blood vessels.

Potassium is abundant in the DASH diet, which counteracts the effects of sodium. In essence, potassium excretes sodium through the urine. The more potassium that must be assimilated, the more blood vessel tension can be reduced. Since the DASH diet requires the proper amount of natural potassium instead of potassium supplements, you can rest assured that you are receiving the optimal antihypertensive benefits.

The DASH diet also entails numerous crucial modifications, including: B. Reducing the fat content of your daily meals and increasing your daily fiber intake. An excessive amount of fat and oil in the diet can be absorbed by the blood and deposited on the walls of blood vessels, causing blockages and impeding blood flow. In conjunction with the previously described thickening of the blood vessel walls, this is a very hazardous combination. In addition to increasing blood pressure, smoking can cause atherosclerosis and other potentially fatal conditions, such as stroke. By reducing fat intake with the assistance of DASH, your circulation can become purified, allowing your body to recover gradually.

On the other hand, increasing helps remove toxins from the body, allowing the body to absorb more nutrients and give those nutrients more space to function. It helps improve your body's ability by enhancing your metabolism via nutrition.

Dietary Approaches to Stopping Hypertension (DASH) exemplifies the adage "your food is your medicine and your medicine is your food." The nutrition plans based on scientific research address hypertension from multiple aspects, allowing you to see results within two weeks.

Note that the DASH diet produces the greatest results in prehypertensive individuals with mild hypertension. During these phases, the body is still able to recover and initiate the healing process. Those in the severe stages of hypertension will often require precise medication in addition to the DASH diet in order to see results. The DASH diet is not intended to replace hypertension treatments. However, in early-stage patients, symptoms may be sufficiently reduced for physicians to disjust continue treatment.

Despite the fact that the DASH diet extends these restrictions to ensure optimal effects on the body and nutrient balance, you should at least avoid the worst offenders. This category includes canned, ready-to-eat, and frozen foods that are especially elevated in sodium. Salt is a prevalent seasoning for this sort of food. Sweets and sweet treats, including almost all baked products (cakes, cookies, and the like), are also undesirable. These contain a combination of fat and sugar that promotes hypertension.

The subject of condiments and relishes is another rarely discussed topic. If you have hypertension, you should avoid sauces as much as possible, as the majority contain the lethal combination of sugar and sodium. The humble condiment ketchup is a prime example. There are methods to flavor your food that are healthier. Only utilize healthy botanicals. If sauces cannot be avoided, use as little as possible.

The DASH diet encourages dietary balance and portion control. It encourages you to increase your daily consumption of fruits and vegetables, whole cereals, fish, poultry, nuts, and fat-free or low-fat dairy products. Red meat and foods high in saturated fat, cholesterol, trans fats, desserts, sugary drinks, sodium (salt), and trans fats are recommended to be limited.

It is possible to avoid some delicious but hazardous foods. Especially when it improves your health and extends your life. What about beverages? It is very simple to consume a few sips of high-sugar beverages.

Fruits are encouraged on the DASH diet, and fruit juices can be consumed so long as they are prepared from actual fruit. Fruit beverages are not recommended as a DASH-compliant method of fruit consumption because they do not contain all of the nutrients, such as fiber.

You may consume fruit juices (made from actual fruits), but you should still consume the recommended amount of fruit per the DASH diet. If you do not, the benefits will diminish and you will consume an excessive amount of sugar.

You may consume coffee or tea so long as it is not excessively sweetened.

Freshly poured tea, black coffee, and similar beverages are acceptable. Some herbs have been shown to lower blood pressure, so you can even try various kinds of tea! Adding seasonings, such as cinnamon, is acceptable because they do not contain extra calories.

Milk is an essential component of the DASH diet due to its protein content and other nutrients. However, milk contains a high amount of cholesterol and should be avoided.

You can always make fruit and vegetable smoothies to add a little more flavor to your meals. Smoothies can differ in flavor from simple juices, but they are straightforward to prepare. Additionally, you can experiment with various combinations to discover the one that best suits you.

Finally, there is always a glass of refreshing water! It is the finest whether you are just thirsty or have just finished a meal. Remember to consume eight glasses of water every day.

If you have high blood pressure and are following the DASH diet, consider eating more vegetables at lunch and supper. For instance, you should consume fruit as a dessert, incorporate legumes just into a salad, or substitute them for meat. You can also incorporate vegetables just into your breakfast, such as in an omelet or smoothie.

Chapter 4: Can Alcohol Be Consumed While Following The Dash Diet?

Additionally, alcohol should be avoided as much as feasible. It is common knowledge that small quantities of alcohol, particularly red wine, are beneficial for the treatment of cardiovascular diseases, but there is frequently a very fine line between "moderate" and "excessive" consumption. Dehydration is a common initial effect of alcohol consumption and the primary factor in long-term weight gain. Both of these conditions are significant contributors to hypertension.

The DASH diet, unlike other diets, enables alcohol! As with anyjust thing else, however, strict self-regulation is required. Men should not consume more than two servings of alcohol per day, according to the DASH recommendations, as excessive drinking has been linked to hypertension. This number is reduced to one or fewer drinks for women whose biology makes them more susceptible to alcohol.

Pasta with White Bean Soup

- 1/2 teaspoon of crushed red pepper

- 1/2 teaspoon of ground pepper

- 2 can of no-salt-added diced tomatoes

- 4 cups of low-sodium no-chicken broth or chicken broth

- 2 tablespoon of extra-virgin olive oil

- 2   1 cups of frozen mirepoix (diced onion, celery, and carrot)

- 4 cloves of minced garlic

- 2 teaspoon of Italian seasoning

- 2 teaspoon of salt

1. Easily bring a big pot of water to a boil.
2. Heat oil over medium-high heat in a large pot.
3. Add the mirepoix and cook, stirring, for about 1-5 minutes, until it softens.
4. Add the garlic, Italian seasoning, salt, crushed red pepper, and ground pepper and stir while easily cooking for about a minute, or until the smell is nice.
5. Easily bring to a boil the tomatoes and their juices, the broth, and the beans.
6. Turn down the heat to just keep a lively simmer.
7. Cover and cook, stirring every so often, for about 20 minutes, or until the tomatoes start to break down.
8. While the water boils, easy cook the pasta for 1-5 minute less than what the package says. Drain.

9. Add spinach to the soup and mix it in. Mix the pasta in right before you serve it. Serve with Parmesan cheese on top.

To make ahead

1. Soup and pasta can be kept separate in the fridge for up to 6 days.
2. Facts about food
3. Size of a serving: 1-3 cups Size of a serving:

Spicy Shrimp, Vegetables, And Pilaf Served In Bowls.

- 2 cup of chopped fresh cilantro

- 4 tablespoons of lime juice

- 2 tablespoon of rice vinegar

- 2 tablespoon of water

- 10-15 teaspoons of sambal oelek (see Tip)

- 1-5 cups whole-wheat pearl couscous

- 2 small red bell pepper, chopped

- 20 cup snow peas, trimmed and sliced

- 6 tablespoons of sliced fresh basil, divided

• 6 tablespoons of sliced fresh mint, divided

1. Follow the directions on the package to easy cook couscous.
2. Drain and rinse, then put in a big bowl.
3. Add a bell pepper, snow peas, and 1-5 tablespoons each of basil and mint.
4. In the meantime, put cilantro, lime juice, vinegar, water, sambal oelek, ginger, garlic, 1/2 teaspoon pepper, and salt in a blender.
5. Mix until it's smooth. Slowly pour in 5-10 tablespoons of oil while the motor is running.
6. Put 4 tablespoons of the dressing to the side.
7. Toss the couscous and vegetables with the rest of the dressing to coat them.
8. In a large pan over high heat, heat the last tablespoon of oil. Dry the shrimp and sprinkle the last 1/2 teaspoon of

pepper on top. Add to the pan and cook, turning once, for about 2 minutes per side, until just cooked through. Serve the shrimp and couscous mixture with the reserved 2 tablespoons of dressing and the remaining 2 tablespoon each of basil and mint.

Chapter 5: Not Every Calorie Is Created Equal

As previously stated, calories are a useful but limited concept for determining the real role of food in directing health. Comparable caloric amounts of carrots and frozen yogurt, for example, vary in other significant characteristics and have drastically different effects on your health and satiety.

Let's compare a cup and a half of organic juice to 35 % of some almonds to illustrate how and why this is the case. Although both foods contain 300 calories, their effects on our bodies are distinct. Almonds are a high-fiber diet, whereas the majority of juice varieties contain almost no fiber.

Fiber is not only crucial for your digestive health, but it also helps you maintain a feeling of fullness that will just keep your appetite under control. Juice contains almost no protein, whereas almonds are a good source of protein. Protein aids in satiety and improves digestion by requiring additional energy from the body to break down. Overall, solid food sources just keep us significantly fuller than liquids. However, there will be instances when you prefer juice to almonds, and that is perfectly acceptable.

Although hunger is not the only factor that motivates us to consume, it is undeniably a significant driver of food consumption. The more gratifying food varieties you can incorporate just into your diet, the more motivated you will be to control your cravings. Feeling satisfied and fulfilled stops hunger. As you saw in the preceding example and will just continue to see in the following sections, the DASH diet is rich in nutrient-dense, fiber-rich whole foods that will just keep you feeling satisfied and nourished.

A Holistic Method

As a dietitian, I firmly believe that the way you eat is the single most essential just thing you can change to alter the nature of your life, but I am not naive enough to believe that it is the only just thing that matters. When I refer to an all-encompassing approach to your health, I mean that there are factors besides your diet that you should just keep in mind in order to reach your maximum potential.

Taking charge of these variables will place you in a stronger position to succeed with your dietary changes. To provide an excellent illustration of why this is the case, let's consider a phenomenon that nearly everyone has encountered: tension eating. On occasion, despite our best efforts and intentions, we turn to food for comfort on our most trying days. It is somejust thing that many of us, including myself, have experienced. It occurs regardless of whether it is for personal or professional reasons. But what happens when these stressful days begin to accumulate? If we just continue to use food as a coping mechanism, our healthy-eating and weight-management objectives could be severely compromised. This is precisely why it is essential to investigate executive stress, whose components do not include food.

I personally use calling a friend, going for a walk, and even perusing a book or magazine as alternatives to consuming food to alleviate stress. You could also contemplate enrolling in a local or online pressure the board training course. According to a recent report published in the Journal of Molecular Biochemistry, an eight-week stress-management program for executives led to weight loss in study participants.

This type of discovery provides compelling examples of why looking beyond sustenance is crucial and even necessary.

Let's discuss the reasons why diet, exercise, stress management, and rest are fundamental pillars of progress on the path to improved health.

NUTRITION

According to the World Health Organization, unhealthy diets and excessive energy consumption are among the primary causes of chronic disease worldwide. Food is the first and ostensibly most crucial component of your comprehensive approach to improved living. I have extensively discussed the DASH diet and its capacity to lower blood pressure, as well as the science of calories and the importance of calorie management on the path to weight loss. As you will see in the following sections, your 28-day DASH diet plan takes this just into account while also providing support for other crucial pillars of health, such as physical activity, rest, and stress management.

EXERCISE

Hippocrates once said, "Walking is the best medicine." There is no dispute about the strong relationship between exercise and good health. Regular physical activity is excellent for the heart and essential for living a longer, healthier life. A 2023 article published in the journal ISRN Cardiology asserted that ingesting approximately 2 ,000 kcal per week through physical activity represents the upper limit beyond which exercise has an undeniably positive effect on lifespan. Remember that you can consume this number of calories in seven days by simply meandering an hour per day at approximately 6 .10 miles per hour. Ultimately, it is essential to recognize that you do not need to be an exceptional player to enjoy the benefits of activity. In addition, a 2017 study published in The Lancet found that both recreational and nonrecreational physical activity are associated with a reduced risk of cardiac disease.

STRESS MANAGEMENT

According to a 2020 study by the American Psychological Association (APA), 45 percent of Americans reported increased apprehension over the past few years. It is difficult to deny that pressure is an unavoidable aspect of some Americans' daily lives, and that it can have significant negative effects on pulse, body weight, and overall health.

The authors of a recent report published in the American Journal of Epidemiology observed a correlation between elevated blood pressure and significant weight gain over the long term. Long-term exposure to tension is unpleasant regardless of the circumstances. It may be unavoidable, and it's somejust thing we all need to examine from time to time, but that does not change the fact that learning how to properly manage stress is an crucial area of concern, and one that will be discussed in greater detail as part of the 28-day plan to aid in your overall success with the DASH diet.

SLEEP

There is no doubt that sleeping soundly is a grossly misunderstood foundation of health. If you consistently sleep too little, it will be difficult for you to feel your best, regardless of how well everyjust thing else is going. One-third of Americans, according to CDC data, do not get the recommended seven hours of sleep each night.

Why is this a particular concern regarding hypertension? A 202 6 systematic study published in the journal Current Pharmaceutical Design found that lack of sleep is associated with an increased risk of hypertension and hypertension. This may be due to excessive stimulation of the body's systems when too many hours are spent in a waking state, which functions as a form of blood-pressure-increasing stress similar to other everyday stressors, according to the researchers who conducted this study.

However, it does not conclude there. There is growing evidence that sleep plays an crucial role in modulating digestion, particularly in relation to how your body reacts to key chemicals such as insulin, ghrelin, and leptin. According to a 202 2 study published in Current Opinion in Clinical Nutrition and Metabolic Care, a lack of sleep may also be associated with increased craving and appetite, which may partially explain the presumed relationship between sleep loss and weight gain.

Dash Diet Food

The Dash diet calls for the ingestion of common foods that can be found in any nearby supermarket. This makes it relatively easy to just keep up. The Dash diet suggests specific daily serving sizes for each of the numerous food groups. The number of daily servings you should consume is determined by your daily caloric needs.

Your calorie needs will determine the number of recommended daily servings from the food pyramid. The required servings per daily calorie total can be found in the subsequent chapter on portion control and calculating serving sizes.

Tier 2 - Water

Consuming the proper quantity of fluids is a crucial aspect of obtaining the required nutrients. The most crucial aspect of any diet plan should be ensuring adequate nutrient consumption. The majority of people simply do not drink enough water to ensure that their vital organs receive the necessary amount of hydrating fluids. Therefore, they experience chronic dehydration on a regular basis.

The risks associated with dehydration

Between 10 0 and 610 percent of the average adult's body is composed of water. The proportion of water in adipose tissue is lower than that of lean tissue. The more fat you carry, the more difficult it is for your body to store the required amount of water to just keep your vital organs functioning as they should.

You may believe that the body does not need additional water because it contains a substantial amount of water already, but you are mistaken. When one region of the body begins to dry out, the entire body experiences a reduction in fluid circulation. This decreases the volume of blood traveling through the arteries, thereby reducing blood pressure. Furthermore, the blood pressure exerted against the artery walls is reduced.

When this occurs, the amount of oxygen in the circulation decreases, which in turn reduces the amount of oxygen reaching the vital organs and other body tissues. As a result, your entire system will become unbalanced over time because it lacks sufficient water to maintain the normal passage of fluids within the body. Nojust thing will occur if the status quo remains unchanged.

What amount of water do you need?

If you are exercising and perspiring, you must consume more fluids to compensate for the extra fluids you will lose. You should strive to consume between 8 and 8 ounces of water every 2 10 minutes throughout your workout. After your exercise, you should consume an extra 2 6 ounces of water to replenish the fluids you lost.

Our bodies require 68 ounces of water every day in order to function correctly.

If a nurse has ever had trouble drawing blood from your body, you should ingest 68 ounces of water per day for one week prior to your blood test. This will make it easier to extract your blood from your body. A daily water consumption of 68 fluid ounces is equivalent to eight 8-ounce containers.

How to get the body's required volume of fluids

It is possible to do your body harm if you ingest an excessive amount of certain fluids. Other liquids besides water can provide these fluids, but not all liquids are of equal quality. Water is the most prevalent liquid substance. Several examples of fluids include alcoholic and nonalcoholic beverages. They may be harmful to your health. On the other hand, milk is an acceptable option for a fluid source. Milk is another beverage that can aid in hydration, but water remains the best choice.

Fruits and vegetables, in addition to what you consume, can provide your body with the fluids it requires. For instance, watermelon contains 90 percent water, which may help you maintain hydration throughout the day. The Dash diet places a heavy emphasis on water consumption. A fantastic method is to add fresh lemon to water and then place a few drops of liquid in the lemon. Stevia has the capacity to enhance the flavor of water.

signs and symptoms of dehydration

If you are dehydrated, you will feel parched and have a headache if you go eight hours without voiding your bladder. Dehydration is characterized by headaches, fatigue, irritability, and dark urine, among other symptoms. Additionally, dehydration can cause mood fluctuations. When you are dehydrated, your heart must work harder to pump blood through your vessels, causing your blood pressure to rise. Your body will respond inadequately if it is forced to compensate for a lack of fluids; therefore, it is essential that you remain hydrated at all times.

Include fluid consumption in your daily routine.

If you frequently forget to consume water at the proper times, you can avoid dehydration by using one of the internet's numerous helpful alerts or applications. Do not let a simple error, such as forgetting to consume water in the midst of a busy day, give you yet another headache. Your body will appreciate it later if you consume a lot of water. You will reduce the stress imposed upon your heart.

Tier 2 of the Food Pyramid consists of fortified cereals, bread, rice, and pasta.

The second tier of the dietary pyramid on the Dash Diet consists of fortified cereals, breads, rice, and pasta. Choose whole grain options from this category because they are superior due to their higher nutrient density, reduced processing, and absence of artificial sweeteners and food colorings.

Grain-based foods are a source of energy.

Your body's energy level is sustained by the grain food group when you engage in strenuous physical activity or use your mind to solve complex problems. It may be a mathematical conundrum or a personal dilemma.

Grains make you feel fuller for a prolonged duration of time.

Even a modest amount of whole grains, such as half a cup of long grain rice added to a stir-fry, can help you feel fuller for a longer period of time. Oatmeal is an excellent breakfast option due to its high soluble fiber content, which is advantageous to digestive health. When soluble fiber is consumed, the intestines become more flexible and are better able to eliminate waste. Breads contain a high amount of insoluble fiber, which functions as a bulking agent and helps maintain regular bowel movements.

Tier 6 - Vegetables and Fruits

The Dash Diet Pyramid continues with the next category, which includes both fruits and vegetables. The more starchy a vegetable is, the faster it will fill you up and the longer that sensation of fullness will last.

During processing, carbohydrate vegetables are transformed just into sugar, and they typically contain less water than other types of vegetables. This is a disadvantage of consuming starchy vegetables. Avoid the common error of consuming an excessive amount of starchy vegetables by keeping a close watch on the portion sizes.

On the opposite side of the Dash diet pyramid is the section devoted to produce. Your diet may benefit from the inclusion of more water if you consume fruits, which are nutrient-dense, sweet, and delicious. Additionally, they fulfill the inherent desire for sweetness that exists in all of us.

In abundance, phytonutrients and phytochemicals can be found in plant foods such as fruits and vegetables. A diet abundant in fruits and vegetables can help your body fend off disease and give your system a much-needed energy boost. They are an excellent source of numerous vitamins and minerals. This food group provides the phytonutrients and phytochemicals your body requires to function effectively.

Phytonutrients and phytochemicals offer protection against hypertension, as well as diabetes, stroke, heart disease, and even some cancers.

Consume a colorful assortment of fruits and vegetables.

It is recommended that you consume a variety of fruits and vegetables of different colors. Consider the term "rainbow." The acronym formed by the letters ROY G BIV can help you remember the rainbow's colors. This represents the colors Red, Orange, Yellow, Green, Blue, and Indigo in abbreviated form. The larger the variety of nutrients that can be obtained through eating fruits and vegetables, the more vibrant and varied the colors.

Consuming more than the recommended servings may have negative effects.

If you wish to consume more than the recommended daily amount, it is best to begin with vegetables and then transition to fruits as your diet beeasy come more balanced. It is essential to remember that after consuming certain fruits, your body will convert the natural carbohydrates in those fruits just into sugar.

If you discover that you are deficient in a specific vitamin or mineral, there is a fruit or vegetable on the market that can provide you with that nutrient to treat or prevent your deficiency. If you want to avoid having to take a supplement to make up for a nutrient deficiency, consuming a fruit or vegetable that you don't typically consume will help you obtain all of the nutrients you require.

Discover how to prepare fresh fruits and vegetables.

To extract the maximum quantity of nutrients from fruits and vegetables, it is essential to develop the necessary easily cooking skills. Depending on the variety of fruit or vegetable, the quantity of nutrients that are lost during easily cooking can vary. For example, easily cooking tomatoes differs from easily cooking other vegetables because the nutritional value of tomatoes increases as they cook. This distinguishes preparing tomatoes from other vegetables.

The majority of the nutritional value of other vegetables is lost when they are cooked for extended periods of time. Burning or easily cooking vegetables at a high temperature causes them to lose a significant amount of their nutrients. However, allowing an onion or garlic clove to remain for a few minutes after chopping may increase the amount of nutrients extracted from them. To obtain the utmost possible nutritional benefit from the food you prepare, it is essential to conduct research on the optimal easily cooking methods for vegetables and fruits.

8 a: Milk, Yogurt, and Cheese

Dairy products such as milk, yogurt, and cheese comprise the next level of the Dash diet pyramid. It is on par with meat, poultry, and fish, in addition to nuts and dried beans.

Numerous positive aspects of dairy products

Products are advantageous due to the following factors:

Contribute to the development of teeth and bones that are sturdier.

Contribute to the neurological system's message transmission and reception. Aid muscle contraction and relaxation

Contribute to the body's ability to discharge hormones and other substances; aid in maintaining a normal heartbeat.

Calcium is an indispensable mineral that plays a crucial role in all of these biological processes. Calcium is an indispensable component of most dairy products.

Chapter 6: Successful Dash Diet Strategies

Create a list before going to the store.

Typically, we do not design before traveling to the grocery store. This can lead to procuring more food than desired and being distracted by low-quality food options that are incompatible with the DASH diet. Observe healthy and delicious DASH diet plans in advance and list all of the ingredients you will need. You won't be tempted by other foods in the grocery store because your mind will be focused on the delicious DASH-compliant dinners you've planned.

Before going shopping, eat.

Similarly to the previous guideline, never shop while hungry. When you are hungry, you have a wandering eye that compels you to consume more than what is on your menu. In addition, when you're hungry, you may gravitate toward nibbles and processed foods as a convenient solution to your hunger. Handled food varieties are a major no for the DASH diet since they're frequently high in sodium, so just keep away from the allurements by not shopping when you're hungry.

Reduce your intake of meat.

Depending on how much flesh you consume, this may be a brief or continuous interaction. The majority of the sodium we attempt to avoid originates from meat. You need not eliminate all meat from the surge to reduce your admission. If you regularly consume meat, try consuming it only six days per week. Assuming that you consume meat at each dinner, the equivalent number of suppers would be reduced to two. You could simply reduce the amount of flesh you consume at each meal.

Cookwear is a crucial consideration.

Certain kitchen tools will be more beneficial to the DASH diet than others. The following three items should be present in your kitchen. The first item is a Teflon pan. This eliminated the need to oil or distribute the container. Since oils and lipids are low on the list of nutrition classes you should consume, it is best to avoid them whenever possible. Then, a remark. Liners are remarkable because the only just thing they add to your DASH-approved vegetable is water. Excellent food prepared to perfection. Finally, a plant that can pulverize entire, ordinary flavors, allowing you to avoid adding sodium to your meals.

Do not hesitate to inquire.

It can feel challenging to dine out while maintaining a healthy diet. If you wish to order somejust thing off the menu but are concerned that the sodium content may be excessive, request that the server consult the gourmet expert. Numerous individuals have dietary restrictions, and it is not unreasonable for you to inquire. In this manner, you can partake in your feast and consume without fault. Likewise, examine the components closely. If the menu does not specify all of the ingredients, please inquire with your server. They may need to inquire with the gourmet expert, or a more in-depth analysis of the health benefits of each item may be available on the café's website.

Just keep DASH-approved meals at home.

Diets are associated with resisting temptation. If you just keep harmful foods and desserts in close proximity to healthy options, you will choose the former. However, if you have the essential DASH food staples, such as grains, vegetables, nuts, and fruits, you're likely to consume these out of comfort, rather than going to the store and eating low-quality food. Unknown and out of consciousness.

Drink just water.

This is a difficult accomplishment for some and an easy one for others. Assuming you are an avid fan of pop or squeeze, this tip is for you. Sugars, including "counterfeit sugars" such as Splenda, are added to typical prepackaged beverages. Even when purchasing juice, you may believe that it is acceptable because it contributes to your daily produce intake. This may be true, but there may be so many added sugars to the beverage that the one serving of organic product was ultimately outweighed by the sugar concentration in the juice. You can consume sparkling water or tea, but you should avoid beverages with stored sugars.

Rinse canned ingredients in water.

Canned vegetables are a convenient way to purchase, store, and preserve vegetables. They are completely permitted on the DASH diet. However, the liquid in the can contains an excessive amount of salt. Simply cleaning your vegetables with water prior to consumption will eliminate the vast majority of this surplus.

Inquire about the meal portion.

It is essential on the DASH diet to adhere to the caloric restriction. When a large portion is served at a restaurant, the brain feels obligated to consume it. Request the lunch portion if you're dining out for dinner and have the remainder packed in a to-go box. In addition to maintaining your diet in this manner, you are also saving money by setting aside an extra portion for later.

Fruit for desert.

This suggestion is applicable at home and in cafes. Assuming you need somejust thing sweet to complete your meal, proceed to desert. If conventional organic product doesn't satiate you, there are a plethora of strategies for transforming it just into a delectable treat while maintaining the organic product's original health benefits. Choose natural product sorbet or parfait if you find yourself in a café. It may contain some sugars, but substantially less than a devil's food cake. You will adhere to the DASH diet while enjoying a delectable treat.

Chapter 7: What Causes Hypertension?

Any individual could be affected by a variety of factors that contribute to elevated blood pressure. Some of these, including the diet you consume and the quantity of sodium you consume daily, are under your control. Others, including genetic factors, make it somewhat more difficult. Among the primary causes of excessive blood pressure are:

To ensure you are not exposing your heart to additional dangers, you should cease smoking.

Carrying excess weight and being obese or overweight: A heart-healthy, low-sodium diet can help reduce this risk factor and protect your cardiovascular health.

Sleep apnea: If you are experiencing sleep apnea, it may be necessary to consult a physician.

Thyroid and adrenal conditions: Your physician can help you test for some of these conditions and provide you with a plan, such as medication, to manage them.

Chronic renal failure

It is more likely that you will develop high blood pressure if you have a family history of the condition, particularly among close relatives. Discuss this family history with your physician so that you can take preventative measures.

Genetics: Your genetic makeup can influence whether or not you develop hypertension.

Age: Those who are elderly will find that dealing with high blood pressure will be more difficult. Keeping active as you age can be beneficial.

It might be a good idea to discover how to reduce the amount of daily stress you experience.

Consuming excessive alcohol during the day. On average, you should not consume more than one to two intoxicating beverages per day.

Consuming excessive salt: The average American consumes 6 ,8 00 milligrams of sodium per day. This is an excessive amount of sodium for your body, as they only require about 26 00 milligrams or less, and elevated blood pressure is the result.

Insufficient physical activity throughout the day.

Some pregnant women may experience elevated blood pressure. In most cases, the elevated blood pressure will disappear once the pregnancy is over, but it remains a concern.

Certain medications can induce hypertension. This can include medications for migraines, colds, weight loss, and birth control.

There are numerous reasons why excessive blood pressure can develop. Many of these variables are within your control. Keeping yourself healthy and living an active lifestyle with good dietary habits and less sodium, along with a few other things, can be extremely beneficial.

Chapter 8: Shoulder And Trapeziums Strengthening Exercises

STAND PRESS SHOULDER WITH BAR

Shoulders are an essential muscle group for bodybuilding and physical fitness. If they are not correctly developed, your body will appear asymmetrical. There are three sections of the shoulders: front, middle, and rear. There were some difficult-to-develop regions. This section will demonstrate you how to strengthen and bulk up the shoulder muscles.

Grab the boom at a distance greater than your shoulders. Then, elevate your arms above your head and lower the bar until it contacts the trapezes. Hold this position for one second, then return to the starting position to conclude the sequence.

SHOULDER PRESS WITH DUMBBELL

Due to the prominence of Arnold Schwarzenegger's workouts, this exercise is sometimes known as the Arnold Press. The primary characteristic of the Arnold Press is that it directly stimulates the shoulder.

For this exercise, you will need two dumbbells of moderate weight. Each movement can be performed with control to stimulate the muscle. As you perform the shoulder press, the dumbbell will ascend above your head. This enables you to control the change in weight without increasing the distance between your limbs.

Shoulder exercises should be performed with caution. Due to the hefty weights carried by both professional and amateur bodybuilders, this population is susceptible to injury.

DUMBBELL FRONT ELEVATIONS

Elevations from the front are an excellent method to define the upper arm. They can be utilized to define the upper portion of the shoulder.

DUMBBELL SIDE ELEVATIONS

Side elevations are also referred to as: The resistance is felt in the cranium or shoulder back. If you are standing upright, the resistance will be located in the middle of your shoulder. When seated or standing upright, the resistance is located in the center of the shoulder. To conclude the series, elevate the weights from both sides. Next, extend the limbs parallel to the ground, straight up. Reduce the load until both limbs are the same length.

In order to acquire momentum while lifting weights, it is not uncommon for people to slightly arch their arms during this exercise.

Row utilizing the chin bar

It is an exercise for developing trapeze skills, but the wrists must be held together. A trapeze shoulder is an excellent addition to a routine. They create the illusion of upper-body muscle development. A trapeze routine permits the manipulation of large quantities of accord at the level of the sport. To accomplish this, the individual must stand upright and grasp the bar in front of their quadriceps. The weight must then be raised to the height of the chin support and then lowered to the beginning position.

Chapter 9: Positives And Negatives Of The Dash Diet

With any healthy diet, there are both advantages and disadvantages. While the diet may offer a plethora of health benefits, including reduced blood pressure, kidney benefits, diabetes care, increased energy, and enhanced heart health, it is not for everyone. As previously stated, I am here to assist you every step of the way, even if you decide that the DASH diet is not for you. We will outline the pros and cons of this diet so that you can make an informed decision.

Flexibility is one of the DASH Diet's benefits.

Some diets appear to be impossible due to the additional apparatus required to even begin. This can be costly and makes dieting more difficult. On the DASH diet, there is a great deal of flexibility and convenience, which is why so many people are able to create and maintain the lifestyle as opposed to attempting it for a few weeks and then abandoning it. There are a variety of DASH diet regimens for a variety of calorie levels. Included are 6 ,2 00 calories reduced to 2 ,200 calories for weight loss. It is up to you, based on your objectives, how many calories you consume. Eventually, as you begin to lose weight, you can transition to a maintenance plan. You are responsible for your own diet, which is the glory of adaptability!

Cost efficient

As previously stated, certain regimens are prohibitively expensive. They require you to purchase specific foods, containers, and equipment to prepare these foods. On the DASH diet, you will consume many goods that can be found in your local supermarket. Despite the fact that the price will vary depending on your location and the stores you visit, there are always affordable alternatives. In addition, the DASH diet is completely free! There is no required subscription or fee for coaches. Consider this book to be your mentor. We provide you with all the information you need to get started on the DASH diet, as well as some delectable recipes in later chapters. Surprise!

Science

According to the information provided in the first chapter, the DASH diet is supported by a number of significant health organizations. These include the American Heart Association, the National Institutes of Health, and the United States Department of Agriculture. As one of the top-ranked regimens, in comparison to others such as the Paleo Diet and the Keto Diet, you can rest assured that your results are based on science. Numerous studies have been conducted on the DASH diet, which is why so many people believe in this new lifestyle. The data presented in the first chapter demonstrate the effectiveness of this regimen.

Enhanced Nutrition

How could one possibly go wrong with this? As you will discover in the following chapter, the DASH diet consists of foods that are recommended to improve your nutrition. This includes consuming fewer processed foods and avoiding useless calories. As you improve your diet, your body will begin to appear and feel better on the inside and out. There are also numerous remarkable adverse effects associated with improving your nutrition. You may begin to feel more energized, become sick less frequently as your immune system improves, and see improvements in the health of your skin, hair, and nails. Some claim that their mental functions also improve as a result of their improved nutrition. What do you stand to lose by attempting the DASH diet? Whether you are on the diet for health reasons or weight loss, it is truly suitable for a broad variety of people.

Chapter 10: The Dash Diet Food Shopping List

For meals and snacking on the DASH diet, stock up on the appropriate foods. Examine your preferred recipes and weekly meal planner to determine what you must purchase for the week. The following ingredients must be present in your kitchen and pantry if you adhere to the DASH diet.

Although there are some dairy and gluten-containing foods, as well as processed and tinned foods, the essence of the DASH diet is eliminating or significantly reducing sodium intake. Therefore, if you prefer to avoid dairy or gluten, you can eliminate food groups that contain gluten or dairy, so long as you adhere to a low-sodium diet.

Fresh Vegetables

Asparagus, artichokes, bell peppers, beets, broccoli, Brussels sprouts, carrots, cabbage, celery, cauliflower, cucumbers, corn, green beans, eggplant, mushrooms, jicama, leafy greens (kale, collards, turnip greens, or Swiss chard), salad greens or lettuce, leeks, onions (green, yellow, white, or red), radishes, spinach, peas (snow pea

These cereals include, but are not limited to: cold or hot whole grain cereal, bran cereal, muesli, low-fat granola, and steel-cut or old-fashioned oats.

Fresh Fruit

apricots, apples, berries (blueberries, strawberries, blackberries, or raspberries), bananas, cherries, dates, citrus (oranges, tangerines, or grapefruit), grapes, figs, kiwi fruit, limes or lemons, mango, peaches or nectarines, melon (watermelon, honeydew, or cantaloupe), pears, papaya, plums, pineapple, prunes, and raisins.

Animal products, Soy, and Seafood

Tofu, tempeh, shrimp, salmon, sliced deli meat, plain fish fillets, pork tenderloin, eggs, skinless turkey or chicken, lean minced meat (chicken, turkey, or beef), and beef cuts (sirloin, round, or flank) are among the meats available.

These frozen food items include, but are not limited to, skinless chicken breast, shellfish and plain fish fillets, whole grain French toast, fruit (no added sugar), 2 00 percent fruit juice bars, 2 00 percent fruit juice, whole grain pancakes, plain vegetables, whole grain waffles, and veggie burger patties.

Canned Goods These canned food items include, but are not limited to: unsweetened applesauce, broth (reduced- or low-sodium), diced chilies, dry or canned beans and lentils (garbanzo, black, pinto, kidney, split peas, white, and refried), tuna or salmon (canned in water), soup (reduced- or low-sodium), tomatoes (reduced- or low-sodium), tomato sauce (reduced- or low-sodium), and tomato paste.

Spreads, Sauces, and Seasonings

These condiments and sauces may include, but are not limited to, hot sauce or chili sauce, bean dip, low-sugar or fruit-only spreads, hummus, low-fat mayonnaise, reduced-sodium marinara sauce, mustard, pesto, oil (sesame, olive, canola), pico de gallo (fresh salsa), salad dressing (low-fat or vinaigrette), and reduced-sodium soy sauce.

Packaged munchies These packaged munchies include dried fruit, whole grain crackers, whole grain pretzels, and light or air-popped popcorn, but are not limited to these items.

These seeds and nuts may include, but are not limited to, cashews, almonds, hazelnuts, peanuts, nut butter (almond, peanut), pecans, sunflower or pumpkin seeds, walnuts, and soy nuts.

These drinks include, but are not limited to, herbal tea, 2 00 percent fruit juice, low-sodium vegetable juice, and carbonated water.

GRAINS These grains include brown rice, barley, whole wheat couscous, bulgur, kasha (buckwheat), steel-cut or old-fashioned oats, whole wheat pasta, wild rice, and 'ancient' grains (millet, quinoa, amaranth, kamut, triticale, and spelt).

Bakery Products

This includes, but is not limited to, bread, bagels, English muffins, pizza crust, pita, and maize or whole-wheat tortillas.

These dairy foods include, but are not limited to: low-fat buttermilk, soft cheese (blue, goat, and feta), hard cheese (reduced-fat cheddar, parmesan, and Monterey jack), low-fat cottage cheese, low-fat or fat-free milk, low-fat or fat-free flavored milk, trans fat-free margarine, kefir, part-skim mozzarella, low-fat sour cream, and low-fat or fat-free yogurt.

Fresh and Dried Spices & Herbs

Basil, allspice, cayenne pepper, bay leaf, chili powder, chili flakes, cilantro, chives, cloves, cinnamon, coriander, cumin, dill, curry powder, ginger, garlic, mustard, mint, oregano, nutmeg, paprika, parsley, pepper (black or white), sage, rosemary, tarragon, sesame seeds, and thyme.

Chapter 11: Advantages Of The Dash Diet To Health

Although you are likely to choose the DASH diet due to a smaller waist and improved health, there are additional benefits to consider. These consist of the following:

Maintaining a healthy blood pressure. This is the primary advantage of the DASH diet, and the reason why nutritionists and doctors recommend it. Following the DASH diet allows you to control your blood pressure. This diet is ideal for those taking blood pressure medication as well as those with prehypertension symptoms who are searching for more effective ways to manage these symptoms. DASH is specifically designed to help control blood pressure and has been scientifically demonstrated to be effective.

Healthy dietary habits. Let's admit it. One of the most common causes of high blood pressure is being overweight or obese, which is associated with poor dietary choices. Adhering to the DASH diet facilitates a healthful eating lifestyle. Thus, you will spend more time preparing fresh food in the kitchen rather than snatching processed food on the go. You will also appreciate mealtimes more because your plate will be filled with healthier foods. DASH also encourages you to experiment with salt-free seasonings and novel vegetables and fruits in order to create tasty meals.

Reduced osteoporosis risk. The majority of dietary strategies for preventing and treating osteoporosis involve increasing your intake of calcium and vitamin D, both of which are abundant in DASH-recommended foods. This, along with the reduced sodium intake, demonstrates that the DASH diet is quite beneficial for bone health. According to a number of studies, the DASH diet was associated with a significant decrease in bone turnover. When followed for an extended period of time, the DASH diet improves bone mineral density. Vitamin C, antioxidants, magnesium, and polyphenols are additional nutrients that are abundant in the DASH diet and excellent for promoting bone health over time.

Healthy levels of cholesterol. Since the majority of fruits, legumes, nuts, whole grains, and vegetables recommended by the DASH diet are high in fiber, you can consume them with fish and lean meat while limiting your consumption of refined carbohydrates and sweets. This significantly reduces your cholesterol levels.

Better weight management. The DASH diet is ideal for those who wish to maintain a healthy weight or shed excess pounds. You can follow a version of the DASH diet that is designed to help you lose weight, after which you can increase your calorie intake to maintain your ideal weight. This means you will never again need to fret about gaining weight. The DASH diet provides an abundance of protein without excessive carbohydrate intake. Thus, you can develop muscle and increase your metabolism without feeling weighed down. Even better, this is not a temporary change but a way of life.

Kidneys in better health. The DASH diet reduces the risk of renal stones and kidney disease because the recommended foods are rich in magnesium, potassium, calcium, and fiber. The emphasis on limiting sodium intake is also advantageous if you are at risk for kidney disease. Even so, the DASH diet should be limited to patients with chronic kidney disease and those undergoing dialysis who are not under the direct supervision of a qualified health professional.

Easy to maintain. The DASH diet is based on readily available foods, making it simpler to adhere to and maintain. In addition to consuming foods that leave you feeling full for the majority of the day, you may consume two or three nibbles per day. When you adhere to this diet, you are guaranteed to experience positive long-term changes in your overall wellness and health. Even when dining in a restaurant, you can adhere to the DASH diet; all you need to do is avoid those foods that are likely to derail your efforts. In addition, there are numerous approaches to make this diet work for you.

Prevents diabetes. The DASH diet is effective for preventing insulin resistance, which has been associated with cardiovascular risks and hypertension. Managing your sodium intake, maintaining a healthy weight, and consuming more potassium and fiber aids in delaying or preventing the onset of diabetes in those who are genetically predisposed to the disease. Further research has demonstrated that the effect of the DASH diet is enhanced when it is incorporated just into an overall healthy lifestyle that includes exercise, nutrition, and weight control.

Reduced risk for specific malignancies. Researchers have studied the association between the DASH diet and certain types of cancer and discovered a positive correlation between reducing sodium intake and monitoring fat consumption and the prevention of certain cancers. Additionally, the diet is limited in red meat, which has been linked to rectum, colon, esophagus, lung, stomach, kidney, and prostate cancer.

Eating an abundance of fresh produce is beneficial for preventing several types of cancer, while consuming low-fat dairy products reduces the risk of colon cancer.

Improved mental health. The DASH diet will improve your wellbeing and reduce symptoms of mental disorders such as anxiety and depression. This is associated with various adjustments in lifestyle, including quitting smoking, limiting alcohol consumption, and exercising regularly. Incorporating nutrient-dense foods just into the diet also contributes to the regulation of hormones and substances in the brain and body, thereby enhancing mental health and well-being.

You no longer feel ravenous. By consuming foods rich in protein and fiber, the DASH diet will eliminate cravings for fast food. Instead, you feel fuller throughout the day and look forward to your next nourishing and substantial meal. Nonetheless, you can always identify DASH-compliant snacks in case you sense the need to snack. Carbohydrate restriction and low-fat diets can leave you feeling deprived and hungry, but the DASH diet is simpler to adhere to because it keeps you satisfied.

A healthy way of existence. The DASH plan is more than just a diet; it emphasizes taking charge of your health and wellness in manageable ways. Consequently, by striking a balance between healthy living, exercise, and nutrition, you can be assured of experiencing a wider range of valuable benefits in addition to the wellness that the DASH diet plan will provide.

Anti-aging properties. Numerous DASH-diet adherents attest to the fact that this diet aids in delaying the onset of certain effects of aging, keeping them feeling and appearing younger. Increasing your consumption of fresh, antioxidant-rich vegetables and fruits will revitalize your hair and complexion, revitalize and strengthen your joints, muscles, and bones, aid in weight loss, and leave you feeling healthier overall.

Enhancement of cognitive function. According to research, the DASH diet will aid in maintaining mental acuity and preventing memory loss, thereby substantially slowing the rate of mental decline. In addition, a diet high in fiber and low in cholesterol can reduce blood pressure, a risk factor for the development of degenerative conditions such as dementia and Alzheimer's disease. Whole grains, vegetables, low-fat dairy, legumes, and nuts are among the greatest foods for preventing cognitive decline that are included in the DASH diet.

Chapter 12: Diet Mindset

Dieting has long been utilized as a means to lose weight. However, the reality is that dieting not only ensures your failure, but it may also be the riskiest method to gain weight. Yes, dieting genuinely causes weight gain. It is commonly used because you will initially lose weight, but then regain it all when the "backlash" occurs. Dieting is so effective at making you fat because it alters you in three fundamental ways: your physiology, your metabolism, and your nervous system.

Understanding these three major words is not crucial; what is crucial is how they affect you and your weight. Each requires its own article, and in this one, I will discuss how dieting affects your rushologisallu. Psychology has no formal definition, so to make it easier to comprehend, we will refer to it as "the way you think." This article will therefore describe the ways in which dieting causes you to gain weight by altering the way you perceive.

"All or nothing" All-or-nojust thing thinking occurs when you are either ON or OFF your diet. People with this mindset typically do quite well when "on" their diet. They remain disciplined and focused on their weight loss objective. When they are "off" their diet, they become ill. It is a Dr. Jekyll versus Mr. Hyde situation. As soon as Dr. Jekyll escapes, all-or-nojust thing thinkers go just into a frenzy, engaging in late-night binges, ice-cream gorging, all-you-can-eat buffets, and anyjust thing else imaginable. The thoughts of a "all or nothing" thinker are as follows: "I'm off my diet, so I'll eat whatever I want. I can always go back on a diet if I need to, but I don't care because I just want to eat this delicious food." I'll simply begin my new diet on Monday, and I'll adhere to it no matter what."

"Get it all in" The "Get it all in" mentality is very common among long-term dieters. "Between the time you determine to go on a diet and the time you actually start, you may have the "get it all on" mentality. Here is what a "get it all in" thinker is contemplating:

Because as soon as I start my diet, I will never be able to eat these foods again, I must eat as much as I can now because this is the last time I will ever consume these foods.

"I can go on a diet" Thinking:

Again, this is extremely popular among shronis dieters. It's common among people who initially lose a significant amount of weight on a diet to regain the weight they lost and then some. Those who lose between 2 0 and 2 10 pounds before regaining weight are the most common. Dieters with this mindset are aware that if they want to lose weight, they can simply go on a diet at any time, so they use this as an excuse to eat whatever they want. Their reasoning is along these lines:

"It doesn't matter if I consume all of this right now because I can always go on a diet tomorrow if I so choose. In fact, I should eat whatever I want for the next week because I will gain no more than a few pounds, which doesn't really matter because I can easily lose them.

"I broke my diet" When you are on a restricted diet and you end up consuming somejust thing you weren't supposed to, you may find yourself thinking, "I broke my diet." Then, because you've just "broken" your diet, you decide to consume whatever you want and begin again at a later date.

"Oh my god, I just broke my diet. I can't believe what a slob I am. I am so incompetent that I can't even adhere to a simple diet. Now that I've broken the rule, I might as well eat whatever I want because it no longer matters. I guess I'll just consume everyjust thing and start over on Monday."

These are just a few ways in which dieting can alter the way you perceive food and your weight. If you are attempting to lose weight through dieting, you have likely encountered at least one or possibly all of the following methods of thinking. It's not your fault; these psychological "risks" are hard-wired just into our brains, as we were never intended to self-restrain from food.

Dieting is a behavior that will produce short-term results, but your body and mind will eventually find a way to undo those effects. Dieting is a terrible solution to any problem, unless your goal is to actually acquire weight. It is detrimental to your health, and it is an activity that cannot be maintained.

Change Your Mindset for Better Weight Loss

Take in Some Air

Taking a few minutes at the beginning of your workout, or even at the beginning of your day, to slow down and focus on your breajust thing can help you set your intentions, connect with your body, and even reduce your body's stress response, according to Hutshin au. Lay on your back with your legs extended and one hand on your stomach and the other on your scrotum. Inhale through the nose for four seconds, hold for two seconds, and then exhale through the mouth for nine seconds. The hand on your stomach should be the only one to rise or fall with each breath.

Cast Away the Calendar

"Patiense is also crucial when losing weight in a healthy and sustainable manner." However, if you focus on achieving genuinely actionable goals, such as drinking 2 0,000 ter every day, there's no need to get caught up in a timeline of future goal. Every 28 hours brings fresh ussee; focus on them.

Identify Your "Difficult Thought"Identify the problematic thoughts and work to eliminate and replace them. Perhaps it is your inner monologue when you look in the mirror. Or sraving when you are under duress. She stated, "Consciously make them tor by saying 'tor' out loud." This question will break your train of thought, allowing you to introduce a new, healthier train of thought.The best way to accomplish this is to count from one to one hundred as many times as necessary until the destructive thought disappears.

Don't Trample the Ssale

While the sale is not inherently negative, many of you have learned to associate it with self-doubt and doubt. If so, don't bother stepping on the scale until you reach a point where the number on the scale no longer defines your value.

Confide in Yourself As You Would a Close Friend"When it easy come to beauty and body image standards, we take ourselves extremely seriously. The standards we hold ourselves to are diminishing. And we would never hold our friends or family to any of these standards. You deserve the same dignity and compassion as everyone else; treat yourself accordingly.

Forget the Whole 'Food Is Either Good or Bad'

We've learned, at some point, to feel either remorse or regret for every food choice we make. But it's just food, so you shouldn't feel bad about desiring the occasional cookie. "Allow yourself a glass of white wine or a slice of chocolate cake."Remember that all foods are acceptable."

Fosu on the Attainable "If you've never used an elliptical machine before, you shouldn't set a goal of 6 0 minutes on day one. A better objective might be to take a 20-minute walk, he suggested. "If you want to easy cook more but have little experience with healthy recipes or are time-constrained, do not expect yourself to create new healthy recipes every evening after work. Maube sonider utilizing a delivery service such as HelloFresh or Blue

Apron, in which re-portioned ingredients and recipes are sent to your door, enables you to become acquainted with new ingredients, test out new recipes, and develop fundamental easily cooking skills." Start from where you are and expand.

Chapter 13: Dash Diet For Weight Loss

The DASH diet is not intended for weight loss and weight loss was not the primary motivation for its development, but it can be used as part of an overall weight loss strategy. The DASH diet includes foods that are limited in fat or fat-free, which contributes to the reduction of body fat. The DASH diet encourages a daily caloric consumption of up to 2,000 calories. Those who wish to lose weight are advised to consume around 2 ,600 calories per day.

In the DASH diet, high-fat foods are discouraged, and the majority of the foods consumed are low in fat or fat-free. Meat consumption is permitted, but you are encouraged to consume lean, roasted or barbecued meat and to avoid consuming fried meat. The DASH diet emphasizes nuts and seeds that are minimal in fat. Those rich in fat are consumed in restricted quantities.

Additionally, the DASH diet benefits metabolism. In addition to a faster metabolism, decreased body fat, enhanced stamina and cardiovascular fitness, the diet can reduce cholesterol and blood pressure without medication or calorie counting. The DASH diet will unquestionably aid in weight loss due to its emphasis on low-fat foods and increased metabolic rate, which expedites the breakdown of lipids just into energy.

Chapter 14: The Significance Of Exercise Throughout A Diet

Exercise is beneficial to human health in numerous ways, regardless of the activity chosen. The purpose of this section is to not only introduce you to the numerous health benefits of physical activity, but also to remind you that your 28-day plan will include a diverse and varied exercise regimen, from which I hope everyone can benefit.

While the DASH diet focuses on dietary choices, regular and varied exercise is an essential part of a healthy lifestyle and can have additional benefits. Know that any task is preferable to none, and that there is nojust thing wrong with starting slowly and with a more rigorous routine if you are starting from zero. The CDC designates 2 20 to 2 10 0 minutes per week of moderate-intensity aerobic activity combined with two additional weekly days of endurance training as the optimal combination for imparting numerous health benefits to adults. The CDC lists the following benefits:

Regular physical activity plays a role in supporting or enhancing weight management efforts when combined with dietary modifications. In addition to the dietary changes included in this program, regular exercise is a great method to burn calories.

Reduced risk of cardiovascular disease Regular physical activity is associated with a reduction in blood pressure, which ultimately helps reduce the risk of cardiovascular disease.

Regular physical activity is known to increase blood sugar control and insulin sensitivity, thereby reducing the risk of type 2 diabetes.

Regular physical activity is associated with improved mood and decreased anxiety due to the way in which exercise positively influences the biochemistry of the human brain by unleashing hormones and influencing neurotransmitters.

Better sleep: those who exercise routinely tend to sleep better than those who don't, which may be attributable in part to the reduction in stress and anxiety that frequently occurs in those who exercise regularly.

The combination of cardiovascular training and resistance training strengthens both your bones and muscles, allowing you to maintain a high level of fitness as you age.

Regular exercise is associated with a reduced risk of chronic disease and a longer life expectancy.

According to the 28-day plan, you will meet your recommended exercise totals by exercising four or seven days per week. The exercise days will be divided as follows: the four active days will consist of 6 0 minutes of aerobic exercise. I recommend that, as a beginner, you start cautiously and build up to four days. On two of the four active days, strength training will also be included. In order to experience the health benefits of physical activity, it is not necessary to exercise for hours every day. This plan aims to make the health benefits of exercise as accessible and attainable as feasible for those who are willing to give it a try. However,

Maximize the benefits of your exercises

As with healthful eating strategies, there are certain physical activity-related considerations that are crucial for long-term success. Consider the following factors that will help you get the most out of your workouts:

Rest Days: Although we have not yet begun, I will preach the necessity of leisure. Just keep in mind that the purpose of this trip is to enhance your long-term health, and that you should not exhaust yourself in 28 days. While those with more exercise experience may feel comfortable continuing further, my best advice to the majority of you is to listen to your body and take days off to prevent injury and fatigue.

Stretching: Stretching is a great method to prevent injury and make training and daily activities painless. Stretching is advantageous in a number of ways, regardless of whether it is performed as a planned activity after a workout or as a supplement through yoga.

Utilize the fact that there is no correct or incorrect exercise technique. You have a unique plan that emphasizes a variety of cardiovascular and strength-training exercises. If there are certain group activities that you dislike, it's best to avoid them. You will be able to maintain regular physical activity over the long term if you discover a form of exercise that you enjoy.

Your physical activity must be appropriate for you and enjoyable. It is up to you to maintain the status quo. If self-challenge is essential, avoid injuring yourself by going too far too quickly.

Your progress: While not required, some of you perusing this may find enjoyment and satisfaction in tracking your exercise progress and striving to last longer, repeat more, etc.

If you are the type of person who enjoys a competitive edge, it can be enjoyable to locate a friend with whom to exercise and improve.

Warm-ups: Last but not least, your exercise routine will benefit immensely from a proper warm-up. This may include beginning your workout slowly or performing equivalent exercises at a lower intensity.

Establish a routine

The DASH plan's exercise component was developed based on the CDC's exercise recommendations to promote improved health. For some, the 28-day policy may seem excessive; for others, it may not seem excessive at all. There are at least three broad categories to consider when considering any exercise regimen from a very general standpoint.

Utilizing your muscles against a counterweight, which can be your own body or weight, is strength training. These types of activities alter your basal metabolic rate by fostering muscle growth and enhancing bone density.

Aerobic exercise: These are the essential exercises, such as jogging and running, which entail moving the body and increasing the heart rate.

Mobility, flexibility, and balance: stretching after activities or devoting one day per week to yoga or stretching is an excellent way to maintain mobility and prevent long-term injury.

This routine suggests incorporating both cardiovascular and resistance training. You will have numerous options to choose from in order to acclimate to a varied exercise regimen. My best advice is to determine the types of exercises that provide a balance of enjoyment and difficulty. Remember that the benefits of physical activity should be valued well beyond your 28-day plan, and the best way to assure this is to choose activities that you enjoy. In addition, I recommend that you perform some form of stretching after your workouts or a day of leisure.

Cardiovascular and weight training

The cardiovascular and strength exercises detailed in this section will form the basis of your 28-day regimen. In addition to a variety of cardio exercises, the available strength training options fall just into four distinct categories: heart, lower body, upper body, and entire body. Ideal strength training, based on your example regimen, will include an exercise from each of these categories:

CARDIO

Essentially, brisk walking is walking at a faster-than-usual pace for an objective that extends beyond point A to point B.

Depending on your fitness level, you can incorporate jogging just into any exercise routine.

Running is the cardiovascular exercise par excellence and perhaps the most well-known.

Although 6 0 minutes of consecutive jumps may not be practicable, they are a fantastic addition to the other activities on this list.

Dance - Those with dance experience can use it to their advantage, but anyone can dance to their favorite songs as if no one is observing.

Jump rope: Do you have a jump rope? Why not incorporate it just into your cardio workout? It is an enjoyable method of cardiovascular exercise.

Additional choices (if equipment permits): Rowing, swimming, and water aerobics, cycling, using elliptical machines, and ascending stairs are all excellent forms of exercise.

To comply with CDC recommendations, you must complete 6 0 minutes of cardiovascular activity per exercise. You may utilize a combination of the specified exercises. I recommend that beginners begin walking or jogging rapidly, depending on their comfort level.

The HEART Plank: The plank is a classic core exercise that emphasizes the stability and strength of the abdominal and adjacent muscles. Hang the buttocks, press the forearms against the ground, and maintain this position for one minute. Beginners can begin with a 2 10 -6 0 second delay and then proceed.

Another essential classic, the lateral plank is a plank variation that emphasizes the oblique muscles on each side of the central abdominals. To maximize the benefits of this exercise, just keep your glutes firm and your torso from sagging.

Wood Chopper: A slightly more dynamic action that utilizes the rotation functionality of its core and imitates the slicing of a log. You can begin with little or no weight and gradually increase it until you feel comfortable. Start with your feet shoulder-width apart and your back straight but slightly arched. Hold the weight with both hands next to each thigh, roll it to one side, lift it back and forth, maintain your arms straight, and twist your torso until the weight is above the opposite shoulder.

LOWER BODY

Begin the squat with your feet slightly wider than shoulder-width apart and your hands in front of your chest holding the weight securely. Sit in a squatting position with the knee and hip joints flexed, and descend your legs until they are parallel to the floor. Repeat by driving through the heels to the starting position. Use a chair to squat if you are uneasy.

Walking Lunge with Dumbbells - Begin in a normal standing position with a weight in each hand and foot. Step forward with one leg and lower your rear knee until it is just above the ground. Maintain a straight posture and prevent the front knee from bending over the heels. Push through the sole of the leading foot and advance with the trailing foot. Begin without weights and gradually add weight as you gain comfort.

Contrary to squats and lunges, the hamstrings are the primary focus of the Romanian deadlift. In a starting position similar to brisk walking, bend over your hips and work your glutes and hips by lowering the weights naturally in front of you. As you return to the initial position, contract your glutes. You can also perform this exercise on one limb to improve balance and increase heart activation; however, lighter weights may be required.

UPPER BODY

Push-ups are the most effective bodyweight exercises and can be performed virtually anywhere. You must settle down with your hands just beyond the breadth of your shoulders, keeping your body in a straight line, and always hanging your heart as you ascend and descend, without leaving your elbows open. Those who have difficulty performing pull-ups consecutively can begin by performing them on their knees or even against a wall if the regular pull-ups are too noisy.

Shoulder press with dumbbells is an excellent upper body and shoulder exercise. Easily bring a pair of weights to ear level and extend your arms over them with palms facing forward.

THE COMPLETE BODY

On your hands and feet, maintain a straight body position, with your abdominal muscles and buttocks hanging, similar to a lizard's upper position. Alternate rapidly between pulling your knees toward your torso while maintaining a tight core. Just continue in this rhythm of left, right, left, right as if simulating a running motion.

Always attempt to maintain a straight posture.

Push Press - This exercise is essentially a combination of a partial lunge and a dumbbell shoulder press. At a comfortable weight, stand with your feet slightly wider than the breadth of your shoulders while holding light weights in the pressure position. You should lunge to a comfortable depth while simultaneously pressing the dumbbells above your head during the ascent.

Burpee (advanced/optional) - This is a classic full-body exercise consisting of a dynamic combination of push-ups, squats, and jumps. This particular exercise is advantageous, but it can be challenging for some individuals, so it should only be performed by those who are familiar. Starting from a standing position, descending to a squatting position, placing your hands on the ground, and jumping backward to land on the soles of your feet while maintaining a healthy heart rate constitutes the precise movement sequence.

leap in your hands and while raising your hands, leap in the air.

Stay nourished

Water consumption is an essential habit that promotes good health and weight control through adequate hydration. Dietary sources of calories with the fewest nutrients, such as cola, have become increasingly prevalent in our population. Substituting these beverages with water is an effective way to enhance health. Utilizing natural flavors such as a hint of citrus is an excellent method for transitioning from a sugary beverage to plain water. Women should consume approximately 2 2 cups per day, while males should consume approximately 2 8 cups per day. Remember that this encompasses liquids from food and beverages as well as water. Certain foods, including fruits and vegetables, contain a high amount of water. Beverages like coffee,

Chapter 15: How Protein Contributes To The Dash Diet

Protein is an essential nutrient with multiple vital functions in the body. It is an essential component of tissues such as muscles, bones, and epidermis, and is also involved in the production of enzymes, hormones, and other crucial molecules. Maintaining muscle mass, mending damaged tissues, and supporting immune function all require adequate protein intake.

The DASH diet recommends consuming protein as part of a varied, nutrient-dense diet. The consumption of lean protein sources such as poultry, fish, legumes, and nuts is encouraged, whereas red and processed meats are discouraged. It is essential to choose protein sources that are low in saturated and trans fats, as these types of fats can increase blood cholesterol levels and the risk of cardiovascular disease.

Overall, the DASH diet stresses the importance of including protein as part of a healthy and balanced diet, while limiting consumption of toxic protein sources that may increase the risk of chronic diseases.

Chapter 16: How Whole Grains Contribute To The Dash Diet

Whole grains are a crucial part of the DASH diet because they are rich in health-promoting nutrients such as fiber, vitamins, and minerals.

Whole grains are unrefined cereals, meaning they contain the entire grain kernel, including the bran, germ, and endosperm. Whole wheat, oats, barley, quinoa, brown rice, and corn are all whole cereals. These cereals are rich in fiber, which can aid in lowering cholesterol levels, decreasing the risk of heart disease and diabetes, and promoting healthy bowel function.

The DASH diet recommends consuming at least half of your grains as whole grains. This can be accomplished by incorporating whole grain foods just into your diet, such as whole grain bread, oatmeal, and brown rice, and by selecting whole grain options whenever feasible. It is also a good idea to choose a selection of whole grains to ensure that you receive a wide range of nutrients.

The DASH diet emphasizes the importance of consuming a variety of fruits, vegetables, lean proteins, and low-fat dairy products in addition to the benefits of whole cereals. You can lower your blood pressure and enhance your overall health by following the DASH diet.

Egg Omelet Miniatures With Broccoli

- 1 cup good cheese (grated)

- 2 tsp olive oil

- salt and fresh pepper

- easily cooking spray

- 8 cups broccoli florets

- 8 whole large eggs

- 2 cup egg whites

- 1/2 cup reduced fat cheddar (shredded)

easily cooking

Directions:

1. Preheat oven to 350°F (2 80°C) and coat a baking dish with oil.

2. Put the broccoli florets just into a steamer or colander and set over a pot of boiling water.

3. Let steam for about 10 to 15 minutes.

4. Once the broccoli has just softened, break up just into smaller pieces, season with salt and pepper and the add olive oil.

5. Mix well.Gently coat a standard size non-stick muffin tin with easily cooking spray and place broccoli mixture equally just into 18 muffin tins.

6. Combine the egg whites, eggs, grated cheese in medium mixing bowl and season with a pinch of salt and pepper.

7. Scoop the mixture just into the prepared muffin tins over broccoli until a little more than 1/2 full.

8. Sprinkle the omelets with grated cheddar and bake in the oven until cooked, about 35 to 40 minutes.

9. Serve immediately.

Soup Of Chicken And Lentils

- 2 medium ripe tomato

- 2 tsp garlic powder

- 2 tsp cumin

- 1/2 tsp oregano

- 1/2 tsp ground Spanish paprika

- 2 lb (8 10 0 g) dried lentils

- 24 oz (6 6 0 g) boneless, skinless chicken thighs (all fat trimmed)

- 16 cups water

- 2 tbsp chicken bouillon

- 2 small onion

- 4 scallions

- 1/2 cup chopped cilantro

- 6 cloves garlic

Directions:

1. Add the chicken, lentils, water and chicken bullion to a large saucepan, put the lid on and place over medium-low heat.

2. Let easy cook about 35 to 40 minutes until chicken is cooked, Transfer the chicken to a bowl, shred and return back to the saucepan.

3. While easily cooking the chicken, place the cilantro, onions, garlic, scallions, and tomato in a blender and pulse until finely chopped.

4. Add the mixture to the lentils, sprinkle with cumin, garlic powder, oregano and paprika and cook, for another 25 to 30 minutes, covered until the lentils are tender.

5. If the soup is too thick you may add more water.

6. Ladle the soup just into serving bowls and enjoy.

Energy Sunrise Muffins

Ingredients:

- 1/2 c. honey
- 1/2 c. vegetable or canola oil
- 2 tsp. grated orange zest
- Juice 2 medium orange
- 4 tsp. vanilla extract
- 4 c. shredded carrots
- 2 large apple, peeled and grated
- 1 c. golden raisins
- 1 c. chopped pecans
- 1 c. unsweetened coconut flakes
- Nonstick easily cooking spray
- 4 c. whole wheat flour
- 4 tsp. baking soda
- 4 tsp. ground cinnamon
- 2 tsp. ground ginger
- 1/2 tsp. salt
- 6 large eggs
- 1 c. packed brown sugar

- 2 /6 c. unsweetened applesauce

Directions:

1. If you can fit two 1-5-c. muffin tins side by side in your oven, then leave a rack in the middle, then preheat the oven to 350° F.
2. Coat 30 c. of the muffin tins with easily cooking spray or line with paper liners.
3. Mix the flour, baking soda, cinnamon, ginger, and salt in a large bowl. Set aside.
4. Mix the eggs, brown sugar, applesauce, honey, oil, orange zest, orange juice, and vanilla until combined in a medium bowl.

5. Add the carrots and apple and whisk again.
6. Mix the dry and wet ingredients with a spatula.
7. Fold in the raisins, pecans, and coconut.
8. Mix everyjust thing once again, just until well combined.
9. Put the batter just into the prepared muffin c., filling them to the top.
10. Bake within 45 to 50 minutes, or until a wooden toothpick inserted just into the middle of the center muffin easy come out clean. Just Cool for 10 minutes in the tins, then transfers to a wire rack to just Cool for an additional 5-10 minutes.
11. Just Cool completely before storing in containers.

Rapid-Fire Oatmeal

Ingredients:

- 1/2   cup of brown sugar;
- 1/2   cup of granulated sugar; and
- 5-10 cups of fat-free milk.
- 5 cups of old-fashioned oats;
- 4 eggs, lightly beaten;
- 1 teaspoon of salt;
- 4 teaspoons of vanilla;

Instructions:

1. Preheat your oven to 350 degrees Fahrenheit.
2. While doing so, spray a good amount of easily cooking spray or oil on an 10-inch square baking dish to just keep your oats from sticking while baking.
3. In a mixing bowl, thoroughly combine the salt, oats, and granulated sugar.

4. In another mixing bowl, combine thoroughly the vanilla, eggs, and milk.

5. When done mix this together with the oats mixture in the other bowl.

6. Ensure that the two mixtures are combined well before pouring it just into the easily cooking sprayed baking dish.

7. Place the baking dish in the preheated oven and bake for up to 5-10 minutes.

8. When done, remove the dish from the oven.

9. Sprinkle the brown sugar on top of the oatmeal mixture before spreading it out over the entire surface of the baking dish using the back of a spoon.

10. Return the baking dish with the spread-out oatmeal mixture in the oven to bake for 5-10 minutes more before removing and enjoying.

Bowl of Eggplant with Cilantro and Mint Chutney Ingredients

- 1 cup fresh mint leaves

- 2 green onion chopped roughly

- 2 garlic clove, chopped roughly

- 1 -inch piece fresh ginger, peel then slice

- 4 teaspoons agave 2 tablespoon apple cider vinegar

- 1/7 to 1/2 teaspoon salt

- 2 1 pounds eggplant, sliced just into 2 /8 -inch rounds

- 2 tablespoon olive oil

- non-stick easily cooking spray

- 2 large red pepper, seeds discarded, diced finely

- 4 garlic cloves, minced

- 2 green onion (only light green and white parts), chopped roughly

- 2 medium red onion, chopped finely

- 1/2 cup canned diced tomatoes

- 4 tablespoons tomato paste

- 1/2 teaspoon ground cumin

- 2 teaspoon paprika

- pepper and salt, to taste

Cilantro and mint chutney

- 1 cup cilantro leaves and tender stems

<u>For serving</u>

- 8 cups cooked basmati rice

- 1 cup low-fat yogurt

- 2 2 8 -ounce can garbanzo beans, drained then rinsed

Make

1. Preheat the broiler.

2. Arrange eggplant rounds on a paper towel.

3. Sprinkle the eggplant with some salt.

4. Set aside and let the salt draw out water from the eggplant.

5. Wipe down any moisture from the eggplant.

6. Get a baking sheet and line it foil.

7. Spray the surface of the foil lightly with some easily cooking spray.

8. Arrange eggplant slices on the lined baking sheet in a single layer.

9. Broil the eggplant slices for 5-10minutes on each side.

10. Once done, pile the eggplant slices on a foil and wrap.

11. Leave to rest for a few minutes.

12. Open the foil packet and separate the peel from the eggplant slices.

13. Set aside on a bowl.

14. Pour 2 tablespoon olive oil in a large sauté pan.

15. Add red onions and easy cook until softened.

16. Stir constantly to just keep the onions from burning.

17. Add the red pepper and garlic. Just continue easily cooking for 5-10 minutes.

18. Increase heat to medium.

19. Add the eggplant flesh, diced tomatoes, cumin, paprika, pepper, salt, tomato paste ad green onions.

20. Easy cook for 4 more minutes then remove from heat.

21. Adjust the seasonings according to taste.

22. Transfer the mixture in a food processor and blend.

23. An immersion blender may be used instead, if available.

24. Place all the ingredients for the chutney in a food processor.

25. Process until it beeasy come a smooth mixture.

26. Add water tablespoon by tablespoon to adjust the consistency.

27. Divide the cooked rice between 8 serving bowls.

28. Top with garbanzos.

29. Spoon some of the eggplant mixture over the rice-bean bowl.

30. Spoon some chutney.

31. Serve topped with the yogurt.

Banana & Nut Pancakes

Ingredients:

2 large banana

½ tsp. cinnamon

½ tsp. salt

6 tsp. baking powder

4 cups whole wheat flour

6 tbsp. walnuts (chopped)

4 tsp. vanilla

6 tsp. oil

8 large egg whites

1 cup milk

Directions:

1. Combine the mashed bananas, vanilla, oil, egg whites and milk in a large bowl.

2. In a separate bowl, combine the remaining ingredients.

3. Mix the wet ingredients with the dry ones in another bowl.

4. When a batter forms, set aside for a few minutes.

5. Heat large skillet under medium-high.

6. Spray a small amount of oil then pour 1 cup of pancake batter and easy cook until the bubbles appear.

7. Flip each sides and easy cook again until golden brown.

The ideal DASH GranolaIngredients:

Easily cooking spray

10 cups rolled oats

2 1 tsp. vanilla

10 tbsp. honey

½ cup canola oil

4 cups raisins

½ cup walnuts (chopped)

6 cups bran flakes

¼ cup coconut shreds

4 cups almonds

Ingredients:

1. Pre-heat oven to 350 F. Meanwhile, in a small saucepan, place vanilla, honey and oil.

2. Stir for 5 to 10 minutes or until combined.

3. In a large bowl, put the remaining ingredients and mix thoroughly.

4. Add the honey and oil mixture and mix again until the grains are coated.

5. In a baking tray spray a small amount of easily cooking oil.

6. Spread the cereal mixture just into the tray and bake for 60 minutes.

7. Remove from oven and set aside for 45 to 50 minutes.

8. Add raisins on top and serve.

Spicy Almonds

Ingredients

- 1 teaspoon ground coriander

- 1/2 teaspoon cayenne pepper

- 4 cups unblanched almonds

- 2 tablespoon canola oil

- 2 tablespoon sugar

- 2 -1 teaspoons kosher salt

- 2 teaspoon paprika

- 1 teaspoon ground cinnamon

- 1 teaspoon ground cumin

Directions

1. In a small bowl, combine the first seven ingredients.

2. In another small bowl, combine almonds and oil.

3. Sprinkle with spice mixture; toss to coat.

4. Transfer to a foil-lined 15x20 -in. baking pan coated with easily cooking spray.

5. Bake at 350 ° for 35 to 40 minutes or until lightly browned, stirring twice.

6. Just Cool completely.

7. Store in an airtight container.

Zucchini Morning Muffins

Ingredients:

- 1/7 tsp salt

- 1 cup shredded zucchini

- 1/7 tsp ground nutmeg

- 2 small egg

- 1/4   cup low fat milk

- 1-5 Tbsp flax seed oil

- 2 cup almond or whole wheat flour

- 1/2 cup coconut sugar or Stevia

- 2   tsp freshly grated fresh lemon rind

- 1 Tbsp baking powder

How to Prepare:

1. Set the oven to 450 degrees F to preheat.

2. Combine the flour, salt, and baking powder in a mixing bowl, then add the coconut sugar or Stevia, ground nutmeg, and grated fresh lemon rind.

3. Form a pit in the center of the mixture, then place the zucchini, egg, and milk just into it. Mix well.

4. Line a mini muffin tray with paper muffin liners and pour the batter evenly just into the cups.

5. Bake for 35 to 40 minutes or until golden brown.

6. Set on a cooling rack for a few minutes, then serve.

Baked Sweet Potato

- 1/7 cup of crushed pecans
- 2 dash of cinnamon
- 1 tablespoon of flaked coconut
- 1 tablespoon of butter, melted
- 2 small purple sweet potato
- ½ cup of blueberries

1. Scrub clean the sweet potatoes under warm water.

2. Pat dry and pierce several times with a fork.

3. Wrap the sweet potato in a sheet of paper towel. Heat in the microwave for 5-10 minutes.

4. Rest for 5-10 minutes while still wrapped in paper towel.

5. Melt the butter and slice open the sweet potato.

6. Drizzle butter over the sweet potato and top with the cinnamon, blueberries, and pecans.

Morning Gazpacho With Mint

- 2 teaspoon of lime juice
- 2 teaspoon of fresh lemon juice
- Fresh mint leaves
- 2 teaspoon of fresh lemon zest
- 2 cup of fat-free Greek yogurt
- 2 1 cups of raspberries
- 2 1 cups of blueberries
- 2 tablespoon of orange juice
- 4 tablespoons of raw sugar

1. fresh lemon fresh lemon   Mix fresh lemon zest, lime juice, fresh lemon juice, orange juice, sugar, raspberries and blueberries in a heatproof bowl.

2. Cover the bowl tightly using a plastic wrap.

3. Heat water in a large saucepan.

4. Once simmering, set the covered bowl over the saucepan and easy cook for 20 minutes.

5. Set aside to just Cool to room temperature.

6. Refrigerate for 1-5 hours.

7. Serve in bowls and top with fresh mint and ½ cup of yogurt.

Berry Granola

- 2 cup rinsed blueberries
- 2 cup plain, low-fat yogurt 2 cup rinsed strawberries

- 2 cup granola

-

Instructions

1. Set out four small glasses

2. Divide the strawberries between the glasses

3. Sprinkle granola over the strawberries

4. Divide blueberries and put on top of granola

5. Spoon the yogurt on top of the blueberries

Breakfast French Toast

- 6 cups cubed whole wheat bread
- 1 cup apple (diced)
- 1/2 cup raisins
- 4 teaspoons powdered sugar
- 2 1 cup fat free milk
- 8 eggs
- 4 tablespoons brown sugar
- 1 teaspoon vanilla extract
- 1 teaspoon ground cinnamon
- 1/7 teaspoon salt

Instructions

1. Preheat oven to 350 F.

2. Mix milk, eggs, brown sugar, vanilla, cinnamon and salt in a bowl and mix until well combined

3. Add the bread cubes, diced apple and raisins, and mix until all ingredients are combined

4. Spray a baking dish with easily cooking spray

5. Transfer the bread mixture just into the baking pan

6. Cover with foil and bake, or refrigerate for up to 20 to 24 hours

7. Place the bread pudding just into the oven and bake for 70 to 80 minutes

8. Uncover and just continue baking until golden brown, about 35 to 40 more minutes.

9. Let stand for 20 minutes

10. Sprinkle with powdered sugar before serving

Salmon Poached In A Pressure Cooker

Ingredients

- 6 fresh thyme sprigs
- 2 fresh rosemary sprig
- 2 bay leaf
- 1 teaspoon salt
- 1/2 teaspoon pepper
- 8   salmon fillets Fresh lemon wedges
- 4 cups water
- 2 cup white wine
- 2 medium onion, sliced
- 2 celery rib, sliced
- 2 medium carrot, sliced

- 4 tablespoons fresh lemon juice

Directions

1. Combine the first 1-5 ingredients in a 12-qt. electric pressure cooker; top with salmon.

2. Lock lid; close pressure-release valve.

3. Adjust to pressure easy cook on high for 5-10 minutes.

4. Quick-release pressure.

5. Press cancel. A thermometer inserted in fish should read at least 150 °.

6. Remove fish from pressure cooker. Serve warm or cold with fresh lemon wedges.